HEALTHY JUICES RECIPES TO HEAL AND REINFORCE YOUR IMMUNOLOGICAL SYSTEM

By Alexandra Cobo (Holistic therapist)

Edited by: Miami Talent Group
Email: miamitalentgroup@gmail.com

In collaboration with: Harmony Healing & Wellness
Email: harmonyhealingwellness@gmail.com

General Production: Adrian Antoine

AF479640

Index

Biography

Hello, I am Alexandra Cobo. I was born in Argentina and raised in Uruguay. I came to the United States in search of a better life. As a Latina mother and wife; my biggest passions are music, nutrition, holistic therapies and healthy living.

Through nutrition and music I was able to find my purpose. I felt that helping others filled me with love and happiness, but I understood that first I had to accept me and love myself, I had to let go of many fears then learning how to love me for who I am, forgive and heal wounds thus to be able to help others.

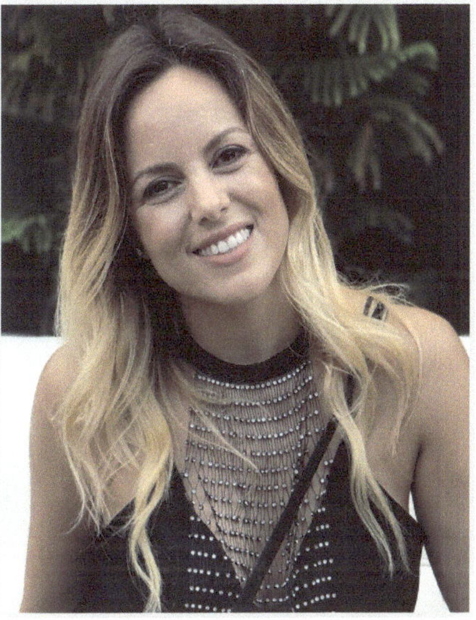

I learned from nutrition to holistic therapies such as sound therapy, Reiki and Emotional Medicine. But above all I learned to listen to my body, that poor nutrition and bad habits could change my mood, emotional state and physical health. I learned that there must be a balance body-mind-spirit, and that's the key for an optimal health.

Introduction

Our body is our temple, we are the reflection of all that we consume. For this reason, conscious eating is vital if we want a high quality life. I'm convinced and truly believe that the Greek sage and father of medicine, Hippocrates was right when he said **"Let food be thy medicine"**.

In all this time, I have looked for ways to improve the health of my family and loved ones to help people get a better lifestyle.

That's why I want to offer you in this guide of healthy juices with my advice, tips and recipes in which you'll find a combination of natural nutrients with medicinal herbs, Ayurvedic medicine supplements and oriental medicine.

Always remember to consult your GP for any change in diet or lifestyle, especially if you have any health problem.

These recipes are **NOT** intended to replace your medical treatments. They'll help you strengthen your health and immune system, feeling healthier and with more energy. They will also clean your liver and colon, speed up your metabolism so that you can lose weight, wear healthier skin, help your body to get rid of toxins that you have accumulated over the years. All of this without having to resort to several medications that make us think we are going to be cured, not knowing that the side effects in the long run are worse than the disease itself.

Natural Juices are for everybody!

The nutrients we can find in natural juices contain a molecular structure, vitamins and minerals that the body can absorb quickly without needing a long time of digestion. You are consuming natural food so you'll feel better no matter your current health status.

To prevent is to heal!

If we talk about benefits, there's a long list of those. Juices clean the body from the inside, they contain bioactive substances that nourish your body with vitamins and minerals, detoxify your body, strengthen your immune system, prevent diseases such as allergies, arthritis, asthma, diabetes, fatigue, hypertension, digestive problems, frequent infections, mood swings, cellulite or obesity and skin problems. You will have healthier skin and even feel more energetic and younger!

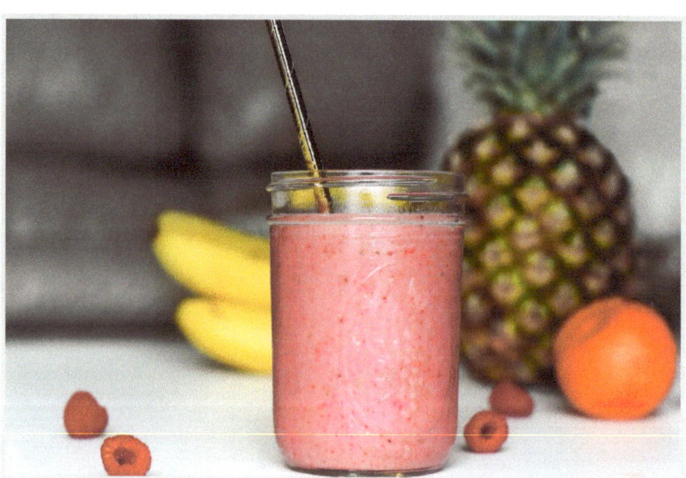

Tips to carry a healthy lifestyle

- Live an active life: sedentary lifestyle only brings problems to your health.

- Do at least 30 minutes of physical activity like walking or dancing.

- Do weight training; it will not only help you build muscle, you will also burn fat by speeding up your metabolism.

- Take care of your diet.

- Start your day with a glass of water on an empty stomach as soon as you get up, it will help activate your organs.

- A glass of water with a tablespoon of apple vinegar on fasting contains acetic acid and has many benefits for your health:
    - It prevents illnesses
    - Balance the pH of the body
    - Improves digestion and gastric reflux
    - Prevents bacteria like helicobacter pylori
    - Decreases sugar levels
    - It will help you lose weight and reduce abdominal fat

- A glass of water with sodium bicarbonate will help you alkaline your body (people with hypertension should first consult their doctor about the consumption of bicarbonate); it also can be used as an antacid or antiseptic which helps calming digestive problems.

- Eat every 3 or 4 hours and small portions, including healthy snacks; this will keep your metabolism active throughout the day.

- Eat enough fiber, protein and healthy fats (chicken, fat acids such as Omega 3, flax or flaxseed, chia seeds, these nutrients rich in amino acids are essential for the body as they work to eliminate toxins and body fat, that it reflects in our abdomen. On the other hand it will avoid you from some cravings throughout the day.

- Eat softly; chew food slowly and in moderate portion sizes.

- Add more fiber to your diet; fiber helps keep insulin levels under control (the hormone that prevents the body from burning fat).

- Eliminate the consumption of sugars; since they are not used immediately as energy, they accumulate in the body as fat. Excess sugar in the body increases the activity of a protein called B-catenin. This protein is directly linked to the proliferation of cancer cells. Thus, one of the most serious effects of excess sugar is the development of insulin resistance, which can trigger diabetes of type 2.

- Reduce the intake of saturated fats (sausages, chicken skin, meats, milk and its derivatives); it increases LDL cholesterol levels, usually called bad cholesterol.

- Increase the amount of healthy fats. They increase the metabolic rate which leads to a greater use of stored fat to produce energy.

- Eat more fruits and vegetables

- Do not consume carbohydrates and fruits after 6 pm, since they are not used as energy, they are stored as fat in the body.

- Hydrate yourself. Drink a lot of water. 2 liters a day will help you with the fat oxidation process and it will help you feel fuller.

- Do not smoke; avoid the risk of suffering diseases such as heart attacks, cancer, etc.

- Moderate the excess of alcohol; this has a negative impact on your health, although a glass of red wine a day is recommended since the grape contains an ingredient called Resveratrol which is a powerful antioxidant.

- Reduce the consumption of salt and sodium in general and foods high in sodium. Replace them with these condiments: pepper, parsley, garlic, oregano, Himalayan salt (decreasing salt intake prevents hypertension, vascular, kidney disease and fluid retention).

- Increase fish consumption (a good source of Omega 3).

- Learn to manage your emotions, control stress and anxiety.

- Sleep 8 hours a day; sleep deficiency has highly harmful impacts on health, both physical and mental, with a high risk of cardiovascular diseases, diabetes, depression, cancer, lack of energy.

- When we are asleep our cells repair themselves. The hunger hormones (leptin and ghrelin) are balanced, leptin is the hormone that inhibits hunger and ghrelin stimulates it, if we do not get enough sleep the balance of these hormones could be altered and our appetite would be affected.

- Practice yoga or meditation. Relax your mind.

- Get in touch with nature. It helps us reduce stress levels, strengthens the immune system, stimulates creativity, connects with the energy of the Sun, activates the pineal gland and balances our 3rd chakra (solar plexus) thus receiving vital energy.

- Moderate your intake of foods high in fat, junk food, sodium, and sugar.

- Maintain a balanced weight. Excess weight increases the risk of developing diseases such as diabetes, cancer, etc.

One of the main roles of nutrition is the balance between **alkalinity** and **acidity** in the body.

An alkaline body is a healthy body while an acidic body is more likely to develop diseases. This balance is called **pH** (Potential Hydrogen) whose scale goes from **0 to 14, 0 being the most acidic, and 14 being the most alkaline.**

For our body to stay healthy we must maintain a balance between 7.35 and 7.45. We are what we eat, so if you want to alkalinize your body eat alkaline foods rich in potassium, magnesium and/or calcium so the body doesn't have to suffer by stealing nutrients to alkalinize the blood.

HOW TO KEEP
THE BODY ALKALINE

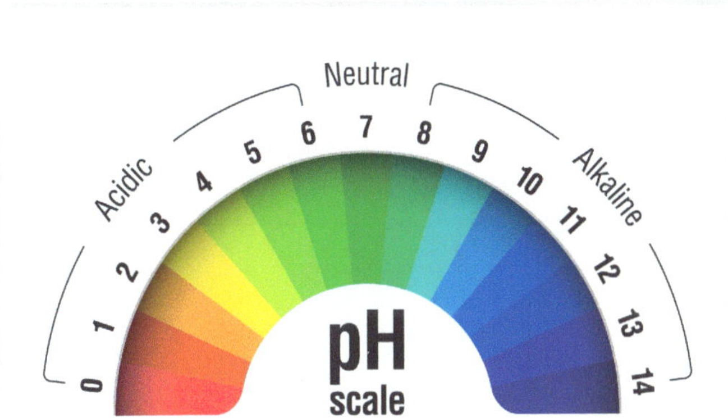

This recipe will help you **alkalize** your body!

Ingredients:

- 1 piece of ginger
- 1 handful of spinach or kale
- 1 handful of parsley
- 2 stalks of celery
- 1 lemon (juice)
- 1 cucumber
- 1 apple
- 1 piece of turmeric

Preparation:

Wash the vegetables, take everything to the juicer and voila!

* Drink it fasting 2 times a week

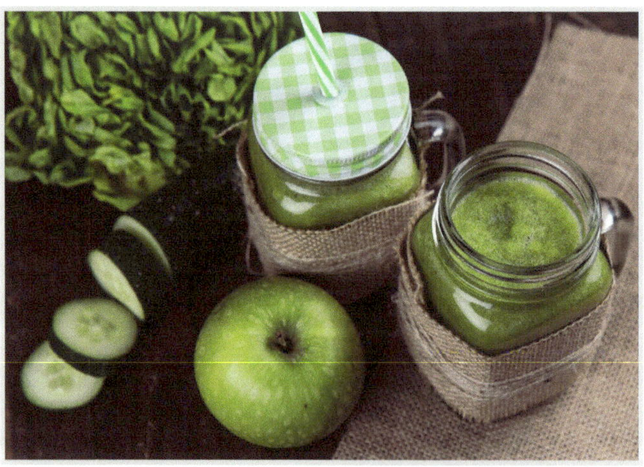

Juice to speed up your metabolism

Increasing your metabolism is the key to lose weight

Ingredients:

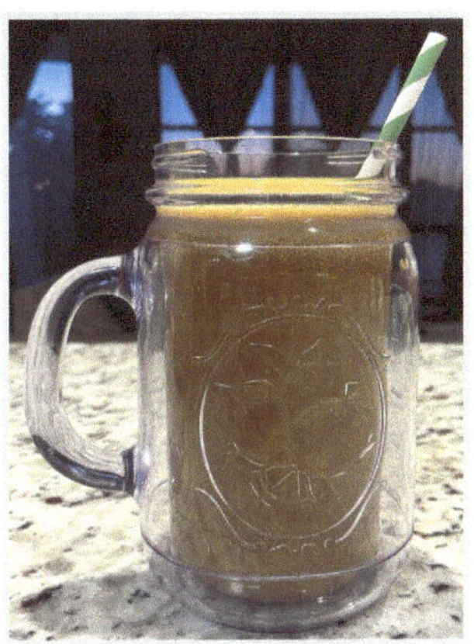

- 1 grapefruit (if you don't have grapefruit use pineapple)
- 3 carrots
- 1 piece of Aloe Vera
- 1 handful of spinach (or dandelion)
- 1 piece of ginger
- 1 piece of turmeric
- 1 tbsp. of ground flaxseed
- ½ lemon without the peel

Preparation:
Wash the ingredients, add the peeled grapefruit, spinach, carrots, ginger root and turmeric to the juicer, then take the mixture to a blender, add the aloe with the ground flaxseed and blend for a few seconds.

* Drink it fasting

* **Ginger** speeds up your metabolism, increases thermogenesis (a process that consists of burning fat to reduce heat and also reduces appetite).

TIPS:
- Don't forget to eat breakfast
- Do weight lifting
- Train during fasting
- Eat proteins
- Consume omega 3
- Take small meals several times a day

Both mango and banana are a source of **fiber, antioxidants, vitamins, minerals such as magnesium** and **potassium** that accelerate muscle recovery and also act on brain activity to **improve mood.**

Ingredients:

- ½ cup of mango
- ½ tbsp. of turmeric powder
- 1 glass of regular yogurt
- 2 almonds
- 1 banana
- 1 tbsp. of oats

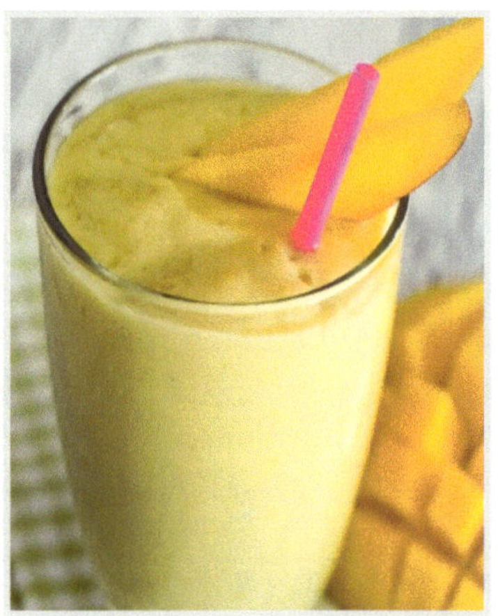

Preparation:

Peel the mango and the banana, add it to the blender along with the rest of the ingredients and that's it!

Carrot and Beet Energizing Juice

Ingredients:

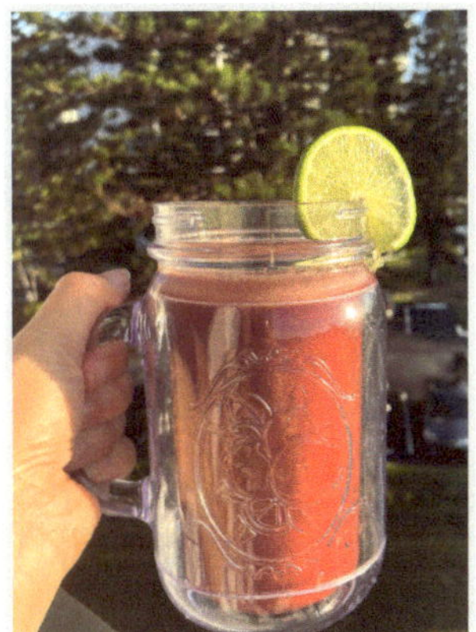

- 2 carrots
- 1 beet
- 2 stalks of celery
- 1 cucumber
- 1 yellow lemon (peeled)
- 1 tbsp. of MCT oil (optional)

Preparation:

Wash the vegetables, put everything in the juicer (if you add any MCT oil, do it in the final mixture, stir it well and voila!).

* Drink it fasting

* **MCT oil** is a very healthy oil from coconut and palm oil; it is very popular among high resistance athletes thanks to its energy source. It helps to lose weight, promotes concentration, increases endurance during training and supports the immune system.

Matcha Energizing Juice

Ingredients:

- 1 handful of spinach
- 2 stalks of celery
- 1 cup of pineapple
- 1 piece of ginger (peeled)
- ½ lemon (juice)
- 1 glass of water
- 1 tbsp. of Matcha powder

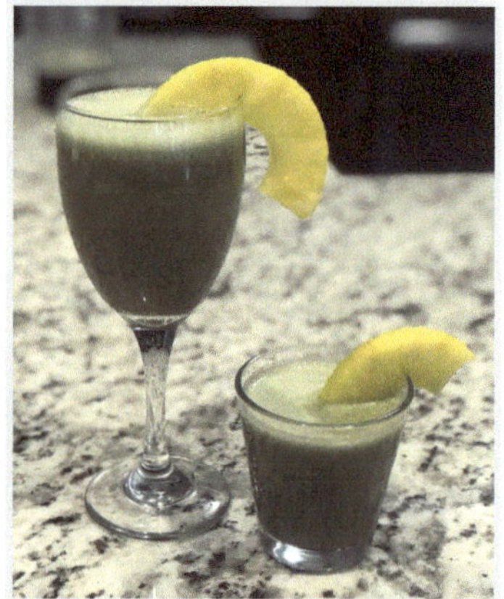

Preparation:

Wash the spinach and celery, cut them into pieces, peel the ginger and take it to the blender. Add the pineapple, Matcha, water, lemon juice, blend it all and enjoy!

* Drink it immediately

Matcha powder is very popular in Japanese culture; it is obtained from the **leaves of green tea**. They are crushed until they are pulverized. **It decreases stress and anxiety levels**, contains **L-theanine** (amino acid), has a lot **of fiber, vitamin C, Selenium, Chromium, Magnesium, Zinc, Chlorophyll**, rich in antioxidants; the catechins that contains **helps burn fat, which speeds up metabolism.**

Digestive juice for heartburn

With this powerful shake you will calm that burning sensation, heartburn, gastritis, gastric reflux or any stomach spasm.

Ingredients:

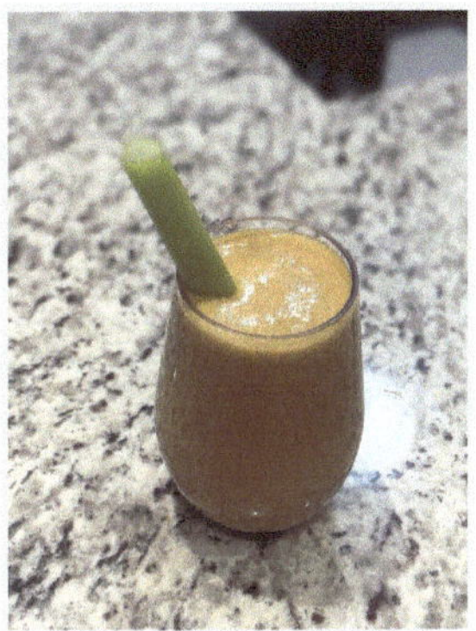

- 4 carrots
- 2 stalks of celery
- ½ cucumber
- 1 piece of aloe Vera
- 1 piece of ginger
- 1 piece of turmeric
- 1 pear
- 1 cup of Kefir yogurt, regular or vanilla flavor
- 1 tbsp. of Slippery Elm (optional)

Preparation:

Put the carrot, celery, cucumber, ginger, pear, and turmeric in the juicer, then put this juice in a blender; add the yogurt, aloe, and 1 tbsp. of slippery elm. Ready to serve and enjoy!
* Take it on an empty stomach or when you feel heartburn or gastric reflux.

Aloe: Normalizes the pH of the stomach and provides a large number of digestive enzymes, helping digestion to neutralize the effect of gastric acids that cause stomach acidity.

Slippery Elm: The bark of this tree (American elm) is excellent for treating wounds and gastrointestinal diseases.

Kefir Yogurt: It provides us with probiotics (good bacteria) that facilitate digestion and improve the body's defenses. On the other hand, **Turmeric** and

Ginger are powerful allies for digestion and inflammation and the **carrot** favors digestion, helping to regulate stomach transit.

Detox Green Juice

Benefits of drinking green juices every day:

- Green juice prevents diseases, gives us energy and contains **chlorophyll** (green pigment that prevents us from getting sick).
- Contains **vitamins and minerals**, is rich in antioxidants, controls anxiety and will help us lose weight.

Ingredients:

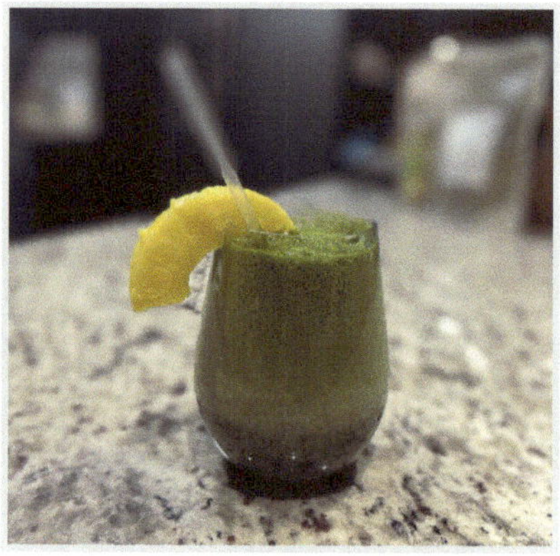

- 2 slices of pineapple
- 1 spinach
- 1 small piece of ginger
- ½ apple
- 1 lemon (juice)
- 2 stalks of celery
- 1 cup of water
- 1 tbsp. of Chlorophyll

Preparation:

Previously wash the fruits and vegetables, peel the ginger, cut everything into small pieces, take it to the blender, add water and chlorophyll, blend it and voila!

* **Lemon** with its high content of vitamin C helps us detoxify the body and **ginger**, an anti-inflammatory root that will help us speed up metabolism, thus facilitating the burning of body fat.

Why is it necessary to detoxify the liver?

The liver is one of the most important organs; it has more than 500 functions, including:

- **Digestive function**: it intervenes in the digestion of food.
- **Metabolic function**: it intervenes in the metabolism of carbohydrates, lipids and proteins.
- **Detoxify function**; cleanses our blood from toxins.
- **Storage**: it stores certain substances to use when the body needs them.
- **Immunological**: it helps our immune system.

The liver helps us remove bad fats from the body, so it is important to detoxify it often so that it can regenerate itself and work properly.

Ingredients:

- 1 beet, peeled and chopped
- 3 celery sticks
- 1 handful of mint
- 1 handful of spinach
- ½ lemon (juice)
- 1 tbsp. of Moringa powder
- 1 tbsp. of Milk Thistle powder or the content of a capsule (optional)

Preparation:

Wash the vegetables, take them to the juicer and then add the moringa and the milk thistle to the mixture. Stir well (if you want, you can put it in the blender for better results) and enjoy!

* These last 2 ingredients will help you to enhance the juice since **Moringa** (a plant native of India) helps protect the Liver, as well as Milk Thistle helps to repair and regenerate the liver and it also protects us from toxins. If you do not have any of these ingredients you can make it with water.

TIPS:
- Take infusion **of green tea and mint with Milk Thistle** in the afternoon.
- Drink a lot of water.

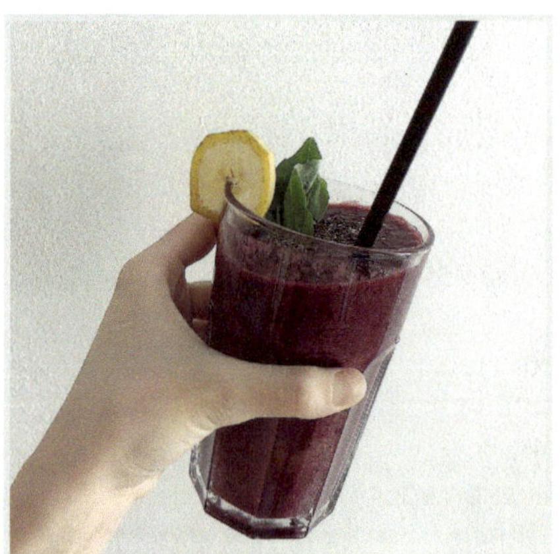

Juice to detoxify the Liver #2

Ingredients:

- 1 beet (peeled and chopped)
- 2 grapefruits (juice)
- 1 clove of garlic (peeled)
- 1 handful of spinach or kale
- 1 green apple (in pieces)
- 1 piece of broccoli
- 2 Brussels sprouts
- 1 piece of turmeric (without skin)
- 1 tbsp. of Chlorophyll

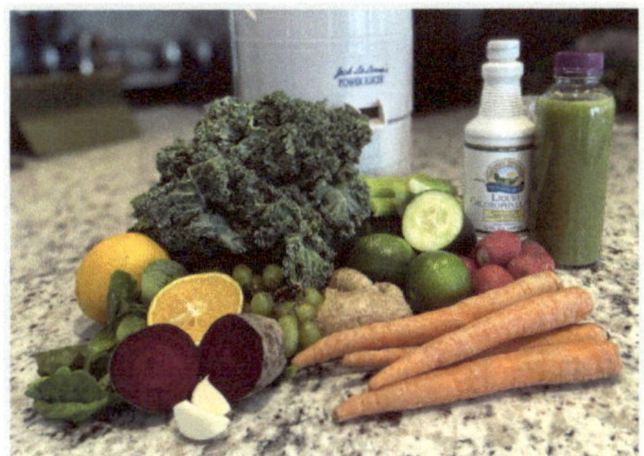

Preparation:

Previously wash the fruits and vegetables, once the beets and turmeric are peeled, take them to the blender along with the grapefruit juice and the rest of the ingredients.

* If you want you can strain the juice through a filter or you can take with all the fiber included or well, use a juicer.

* Take it while fasting for 9 days and rest.

* Chlorophyll is a green pigment found in the leaves, stems of some plants and various algae, it has many health benefits, keeps our digestive system healthy, protects the liver, stomach and gallbladder, reinforces memory, balances blood glucose levels, improves circulation among others.

TIPS: drink curcuma tea and boldo during the afternoons.

Juice to detoxify the kidneys

The kidneys are one of the most important organs since they are in charge of filtering and detoxifying the body. They eliminate the acid produced by the body's cells, maintaining a healthy balance of water, salts and minerals in the blood.

Signs of kidneys malfunction:

Changes in urination and appearance of the urine, fluid retention, tiredness and fatigue, anemia and vomiting.

Here is an excellent recipe to clean your kidney!

Ingredients:

- 1 whole pineapple
- 1 whole celery (cut the base)
- 1 handful of coriander
- 1 handful of parsley
- 1 handful of dandelions

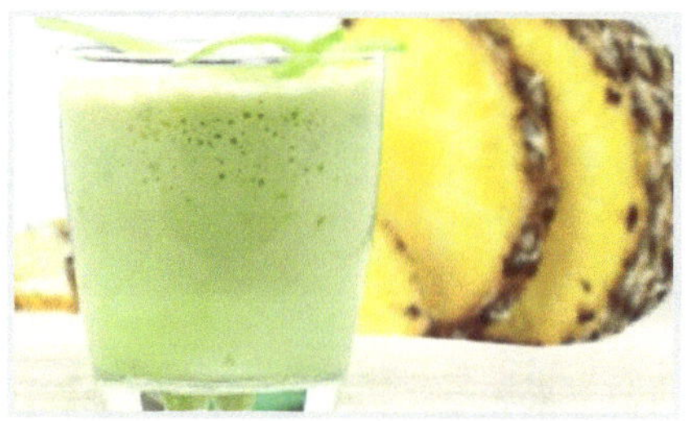

Preparation:

Wash all the ingredients, peel the pineapple, cut it into pieces and take it to the juicer along with the rest of the ingredients.
* Take on an empty stomach and in mid-afternoon, 2 hours before or after a meal.

TIPS:
- Drink plenty of water, if possible lemon water
- Eat antioxidant fruits (blueberry, blackberry and cranberry)
- Eat celery, omega 3 and take multivitamins
- Consume vitamin B6 and stone breaker infusions.

What are the functions of the pancreas?

The pancreas is the organ that filters waste produced in the body. If it accumulates a lot of toxins, it won't be able to function properly. It produces insulin and also many other enzymes that are essential for the digestion process.

Ingredients:

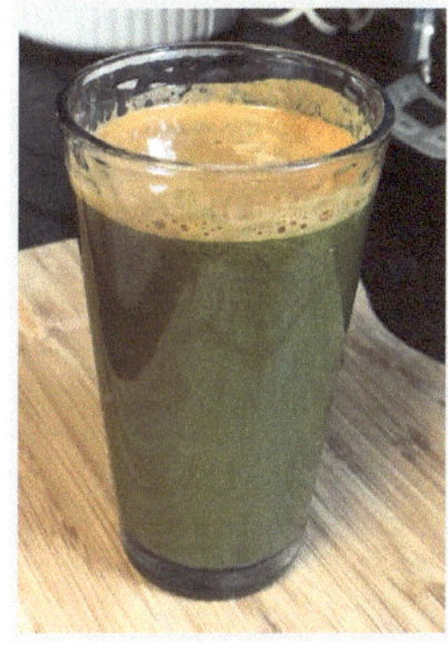

- 1 piece of aloe
- 2 carrots
- 1 handful of spinach
- 2 Brussels sprouts
- 1 piece of Nopal
- 1 piece of celery
- 1 glass of water

Preparation:

Wash the vegetables, peel the aloe, cut the carrots into pieces and put everything in the blender, blend and voila!

*If you want you can strain the fiber or take it with all the pulp.
*Take it 1 to 3 times a day separated from meals for 7 days and rest.

The **Nopal** is rich in soluble fibers; it has a satiety effect and reduces fat absorption at the intestinal level, which contributes to weight loss. In addition, the nopal plant fibers control the excess production of gastric acid and protect the mucosa of the stomach and intestines.

Ingredients:

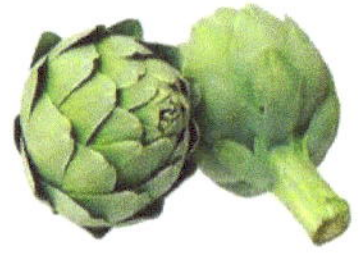

- 1 cup of papaya
- 1 tbsp. Of flaxseed (seeds or ground)
- 4 to 6 almonds
- 1 cup artichoke water (cold infusion)

Preparation:

Peel and cut the papaya and remove the seeds. Put everything in the blender and add the artichoke water (make sure it's cold). Blend for 60 seconds and drink as soon as possible.

* You can drink it every morning.

TIPS:
- Do not throw away the papaya seeds; they are useful to detoxify the liver, kidneys and digestive system.
- Consume the following ingredients:
- dandelion, garlic, Echinacea, gentian root, cinnamon and ginger.

Artichokes purify our body of toxins; take care of our pancreas, liver and also the gallbladder. And Papaya promotes digestion and reduces inflammation.

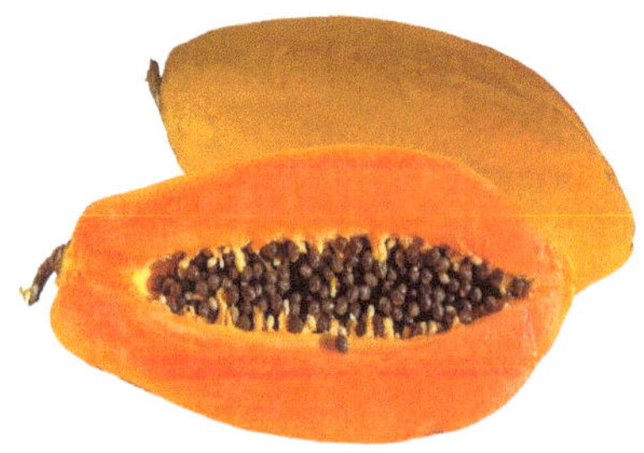

Ingredients:

- 1 cup of broccoli
- 1 cup of cauliflower
- ½ cucumber
- 2 carrots
- ½ glass of water

Preparation:

Wash all the vegetables and take everything to the juicer, transfer the contents to a jug and then add the water.

* Take in the morning at natural temperature and take it warm at night. For 10 days, rest 20 days (detoxify 3 times a year)

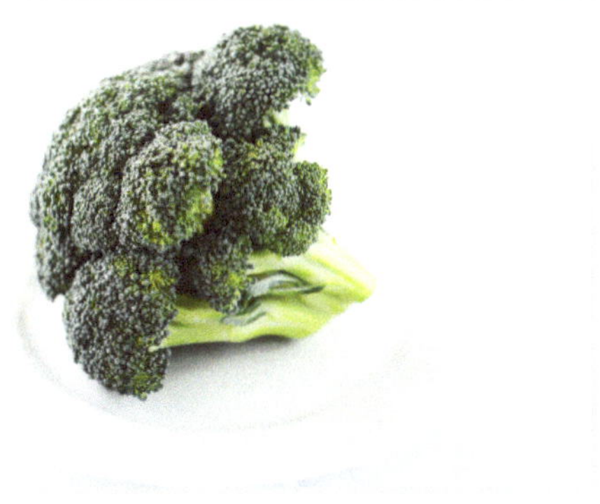

Juice to detoxify the blood #1

Our body requires optimal oxygenation and nutrients supply through the blood. When the blood is not in an adequate state, some disorders may occur due to imbalance, such as allergies, skin problems, continuous colds, etc.

Ingredients:

- 1 large or 2 small beets
- 8 oz. of grapes
- 1 tbsp. Of chlorophyll
- 1 handful of dandelions

Preparation:

Wash the fruits and vegetables, cut the beets in half and put everything to the juicer, then add the chlorophyll to the rest of the juice and stir well, and voila!

* Take it while fasting.

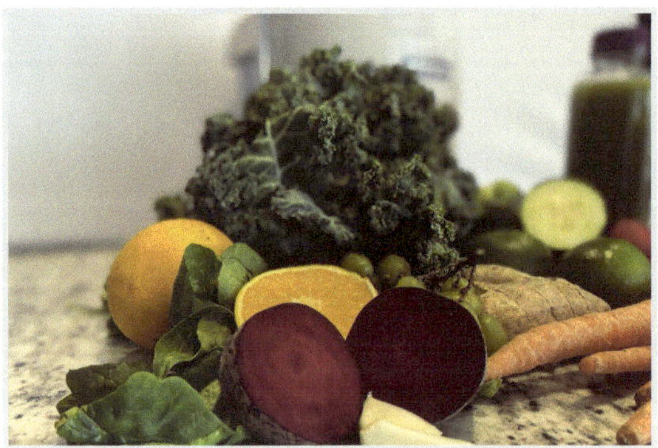

Juice to detoxify the blood #2

Ingredients:

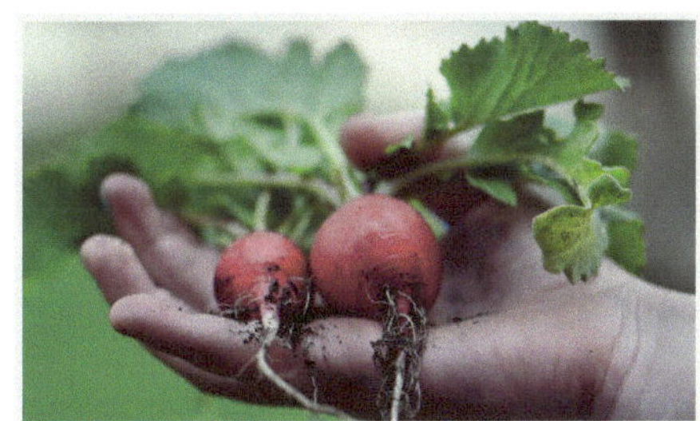

- 3 stalks of celery
- 10 radishes
- 1 lemon without peel
- 1 tbsp. of chlorella powder
- 1 tbsp. of honey

Preparation:

Wash the celery and radishes, bring them to the juicer with the lemon after removing the peel and add the tbsp. of chlorella and honey to the final mixture and stir well.

* Take it on an empty stomach

Chlorella is an alga with a great source of protein that contains essential minerals and amino acids. Due to its high content of antioxidants, chlorophyll helps to oxygenate the blood avoiding cardiovascular diseases. It is a purifying alga for the body that provides large doses of vitamin B12, perfect for vegetarians and vegans looking for proteins and vitamins that are not from animal sources.

TIPS:
It helps purify the blood with these nutrients:
Omega 3 and omega 6, amaranth (from India), whole grains, seeds, nuts, vitamin C, lemon, onion and foods rich in vitamin A like carrots.

Juice to strengthen the immune system #1

The importance of strengthening our immune system:

The immune system is a natural defense system of the organism against infections, bacteria and viruses. It reacts by secreting antibodies and destroying the infectious organisms that invade. When our system is weakened it cannot defend itself against these antibodies and viruses and therefore we end up getting sick.

This is one of my favorite recipes to strengthen the immune system!

Ingredients:

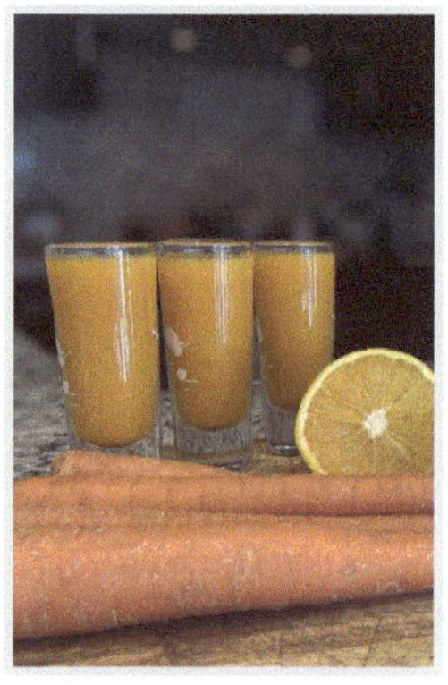

- 3 large carrots
- 3 oranges
- 1 small piece of ginger
- 1/2 yellow lemon
- 1 glass of coconut water
- 1 tbsp. of turmeric (powder or root)
- 1 little black pepper

Preparation:

Wash the carrots and ginger, peel the oranges and the lemon, bring everything to the juicer and put the final mixture in a jar. Add the coconut water and turmeric powder. You can also use a blender to better mix the nutrients.

* Take it on an empty stomach or mid-afternoon, 1 or 2 hours before or after each meal.

TIPS:

These medicinal plants will help you strengthen your system and prevent viral infections: Echinacea - Astragalus - Elderberry

Juice to strengthen the immune system #2

Ingredients:

- 1 large or 2 small beets
- 3 carrots
- 1 piece of ginger
- 1 piece of turmeric or ½ tbsp. of turmeric powdered
- ½ tbsp. of elderberry powder (optional)

Preparation:

Wash the vegetables, cut the beets in half and bring them to the juicer along with the carrot, ginger root and turmeric root (if the turmeric is in powder, then add it after to the mixture and mix well). Serve, add the elderberry powder, stir the juice well and enjoy!

* Drink it as soon as possible.

* **Elderberry**: is a medicinal plant that has great health benefits. It not only strengthens the immune system, it is also effective against viruses, colds and flu. It's high in flavonoids "rich in antioxidants", fiber, vitamin A, vitamin B6, iron, potassium, beta-carotene, it has 87% more vitamin C than any other plant!

* Some doctors do NOT recommend consuming this plant to pregnant or lactating women.

Antiviral juice

Did you know?

Hot pepper has high levels of vitamin C, beta-carotenes. It also relaxes blood vessels, contains **capsaicin** which prevents sinusitis and congestion, and eliminates bacteria from the stomach and produces endorphins (the hormone of well-being).

Ingredients:

- 1 whole pineapple
- 1 bundle of celery
- 3 oranges
- 2 hot red or yellow chili peppers (or 1 garlic)
- 1 ginger root

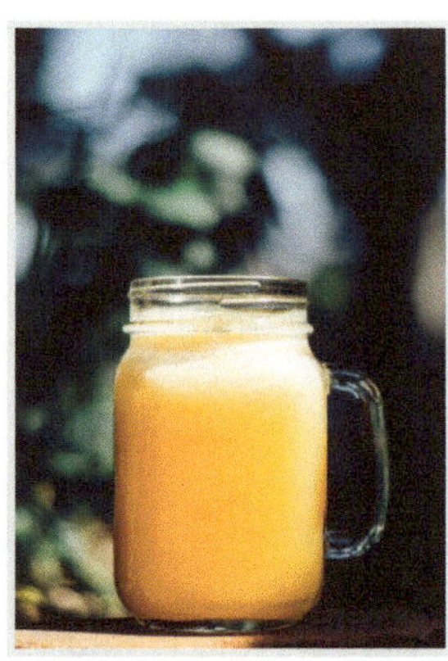

Preparation:

(To disinfect fruits and vegetables of pesticides, soak them for a few minutes with water and a few drops of white vinegar).

Wash all the fruits and vegetables; peel the oranges and the pineapple. Bring everything to the juicer with the rest of the ingredients and that's it!

* Take it early in the morning and between meals in the afternoon.

TIPS:
Consume lemon, onion, garlic, echinacea and astragalus.

Anti-inflammatory juice #1

Inflammation is a natural autoimmune response of the body. It's a symptom of stress inside our body indicating that something is wrong. When an external element such as bacteria or viruses and toxins enters our body, it reacts by attacking with inflammation.

Ingredients:

- 1 whole pineapple
- 1 large handful of kale
- 1 piece of ginger root
- 1 piece of turmeric root

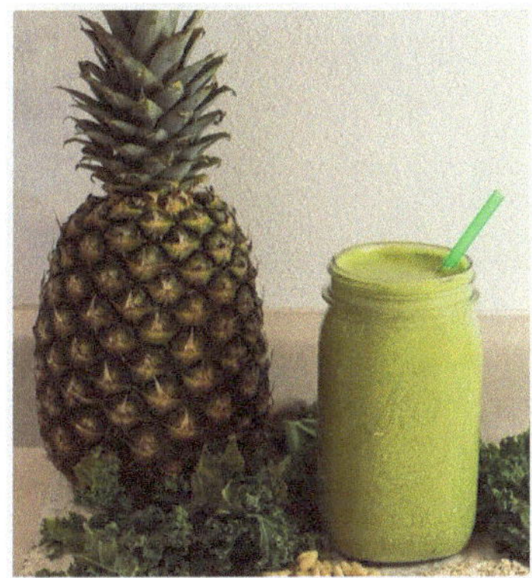

Preparation:

Peel the pineapple, cut it into pieces and wash everything, then take all the ingredients to the juicer.

* Take right away, preferably in the morning or mid-afternoon between meals.

Anti-inflammatory juice 2

Ingredients:

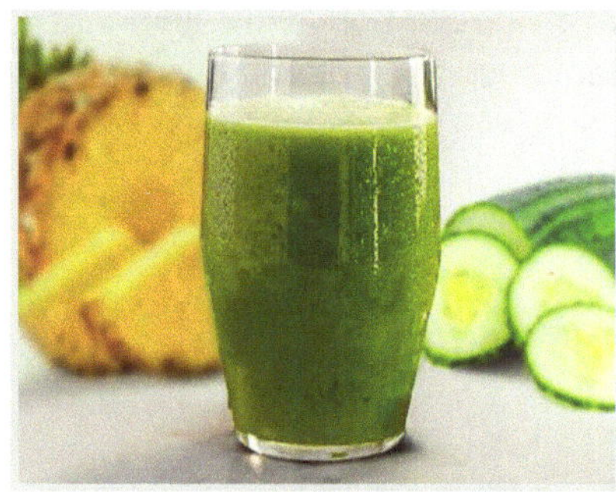

- 1 cup of pineapple
- 1 cucumber
- 1 piece of ginger (peeled)
- 1 lemon (juice)
- 1 glass of water

Preparation:

Wash all the ingredients, peel and cut the pineapple into pieces, chop the cucumber, peel the ginger, take everything to the blender, add the lemon juice and the water. Enjoy!

* Take it as soon as possible

TIPS:
Foods that promote inflammation:
Processed foods, refined flours and sugars, milk and its derivatives, red meat, cereals with gluten and vegetable oil.

Anti-inflammatory foods:
Turmeric, ginger, chia seeds, green leafy vegetables, cruciferous (cabbages and broccoli) probiotics, fruits such as blueberries, blackberries and strawberries.

Anti-cancer juice #1

Ingredients:

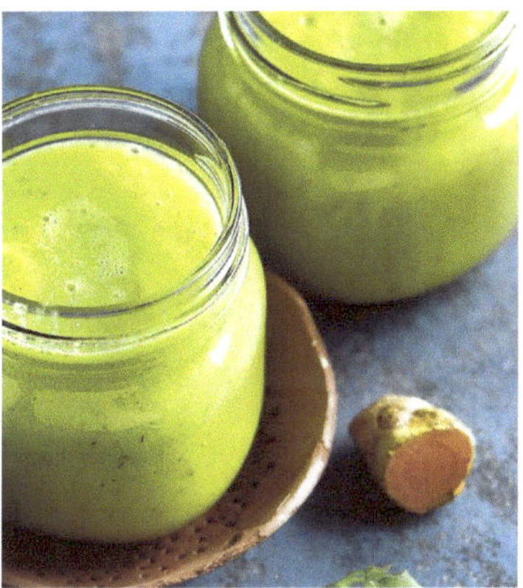

- 1 apple
- 2 stalks of celery
- 1 turmeric root
- 1 lemon (juice)
- 1 handful of Kale (or dandelion)
- 1 cucumber
- 1 tbsp. of honey

Preparation:

Wash everything beforehand, take everything to the juicer (except honey) and serve!
* Take it for three weeks.

TIPS:

Consume infusions of green tea, Oolong tea, and medicinal mushrooms like Reishi (ganoderma)

Anti-cancer juice #2

Ingredients:

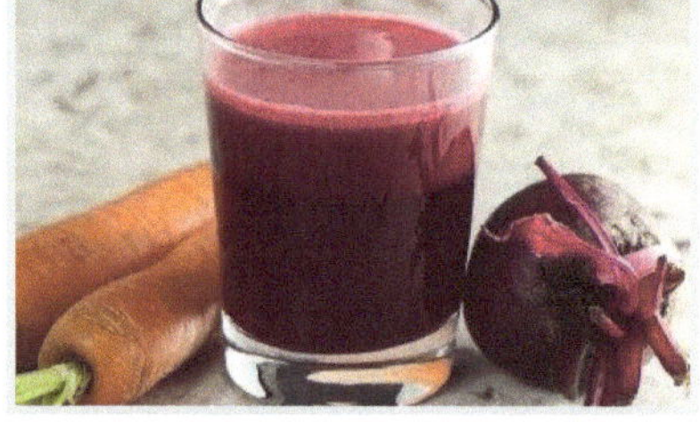

- 1 large beet or 2 small beets
- 1 cup of grapes
- 1 cup of berries (blueberries, blackberries, raspberries)
- 1 lemon without peel
- 2 carrots

Preparation:

Wash the ingredients beforehand, chop it into small pieces and take everything to the juicer, except the lemon juice. Add it last (you can use a blender adding a glass of water).

* Take on an empty stomach

Did you know?

Grapes, as well as red wine, contain a large amount of antioxidants called **resveratrol**. This powerful antioxidant reduces the risk of contracting prostate cancer by 50%, reducing the levels of male hormones such as testosterone.

TIPS:

Eat broccoli and cauliflower. They are vegetables with high anticancer properties, like green tea, mushrooms, pure cocoa, red berries, garlic, olive oil, nuts, red wine; its content of **polyphenols** and **tannins** makes it a great ally thanks to its antioxidant power. Ginger and turmeric also have very good anti-cancer properties.

Antioxidant juice

Antioxidants help protect the body against the formation of **free radicals**. These **free radicals** are atoms that cause damage to the cell, deteriorating the immune system and contracting infections and diseases.

Ingredients:

- 1 cup of raspberry
- 1 cup of strawberries
- 1 cup of cranberry
- 1 cup of blueberries
- 1 tbsp. of chia seeds
- 1 glass of water

Preparation:

Wash all the fruits beforehand and put it in the blender, then put the chia seeds in the glass of water, let them rest for a few minutes and stir it. Finally take it to the blender, blend and enjoy!

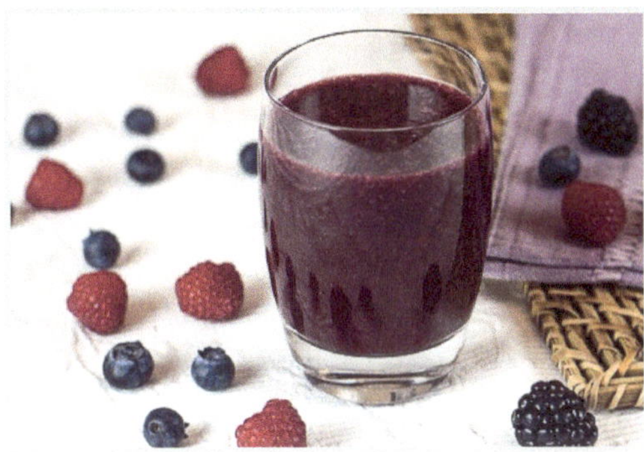

Ingredients:

- 4 stalks of celery
- 4 pineapple slices
- 1 glass of coconut water

Preparation:

Wash the fruits and vegetables, put everything in the blender and blend.

* Take it right away

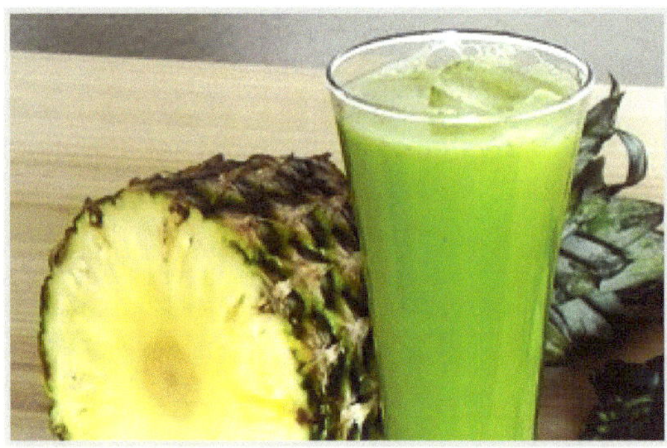

Rejuvenating juice

Ingredients:

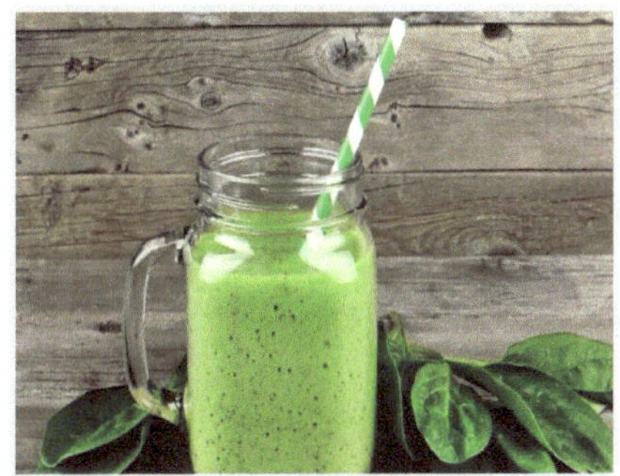

- 1 cucumber
- 1 apple
- 1 handful of spinach
- 4 stalks of celery

Preparation:

Wash all the ingredients and take them to the juicer, in case of using a blender add a glass of water and enjoy!

* You can drink it in the mornings or after 2 hours between meals.

TIPS:
Drink a lot of water
Don't abuse makeup, the pores need to breathe!
Don't abuses of the sun, always try to use sunscreen
even when you go for a walk.
Get used to having healthy habits.
Eat plenty of fruit and vegetables.

Why is it important to cleanse the colon?

The colon is responsible for eliminating toxins and waste, a good colon cleansing will improve your health by eliminating those toxins, increasing energy, improving the immune system and preventing diseases.

Ingredients:

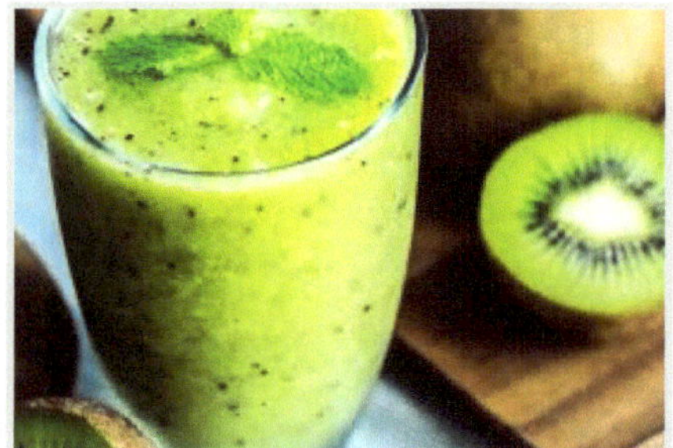

- ½ lemon
- 1 kiwi
- 1 apple
- 1 stalk of celery
- 1 tbsp. of chia seed
- 1 glass of water

Preparation:

Wash the ingredients, cut them into pieces and put the chia seeds in the glass with water, let them rest for 5 minutes and stir, then put everything in the blender and blend.

* Take it on an empty stomach

Juice to cleanse the colon #2

Ingredients:

- 2 stalk of celery
- 2 slices of pineapple
- 2 prickly pear cactus (without thorns)
- 1 tbsp. of ground flaxseed
- 1 cup of water (if you want more liquid you can add a little more water)

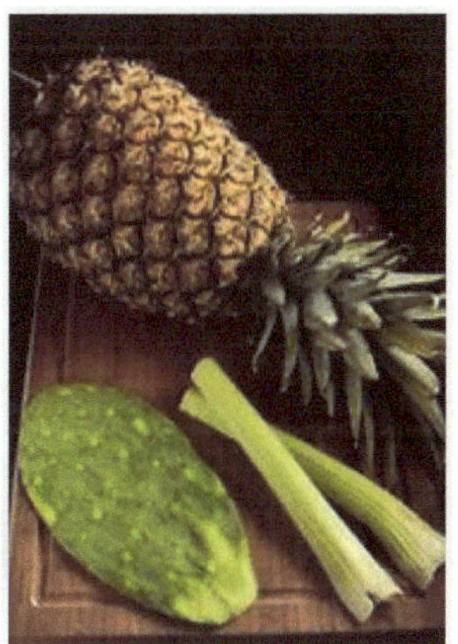

Preparation:

Wash the celery and the nopal. Remove the spines from the nopal and cut it into pieces, bring everything to the blender together with the pineapple, water, linseed and blend.

* Take it on an empty stomach

The Nopal: favors digestion due to its rich soluble fiber, it has a satiety effect and reduces fat absorption at the intestinal level, contributing to weight reduction, also beneficial for diabetes, osteoporosis. It is also an antioxidant and anti-cancer.

The 7 Chakras

Did you know that what you eat could help align your chakras?

What are chakras?

The chakras are energy centers of the body through which the life force and the vital energy flows.

According to the Hindu culture, there are many chakras and energy points throughout the body, but there are 7 main ones and they are located along the axis of the spine. Each chakra encompasses different organs of the body, when these chakras are blocked, vital energy doesn't flow.

Imagine a pipe tube that was blocked; the water wouldn't flow correctly, right? Well, it is the same with these energy points. When they are blocked, we experience mood swings, discomfort in certain parts of the body and the organs related to those chakras begin to show that something is wrong, such as allergies, chronic inflammation, and illnesses that we could relate to a imbalanced organ in disharmony.

Chakras: their colors, organs, related pathologies and foods that benefit them

 physical support of the body.

Spinal base, legs, bones, feet, rectum (chronic lower back pain, sciatica and varicose veins)

Eat protein, tubers, and red foods like pomegranates, strawberries, raspberry and beets.

: sexual organs.

Large intestine, bladder, hips, pelvis (chronic pain in the lower back, pelvic pain, sexual potency, reproductive organs, urinary problems).

* In this chakra lie our decisions and also fears

To align them you can consume: healthy fats, fish, orange-colored foods such as carrots and peaches.

: abdomen and stomach

Small intestine, gallbladder, kidneys, pancreas, adrenal glands, spleen, central part of the spine (gastric ulcers, pancreatitis, diabetes, chronic or acute indigestion, anorexia, bulimia, liver dysfunction and hepatitis).

All our emotions, fears, joys, sadness and also our personal power are contained here.

Food: carbohydrates, whole grains, legumes, yellow foods like corn, banana, and pineapple.

4th Heart Chakra: heart and circulatory system

Lungs, shoulders, arms, ribs, chest, diaphragm (heart failure, asthma, allergy, pneumonia, lung cancer, upper back and breast cancer).

* The way we relate, the way I love myself and the way they love me.

Food: vegetables, fruits and green leafy vegetables, foods rich in chlorophyll, etc.

5th Throat Chakra: Thyroid, trachea, cervical vertebrae, mouth, teeth and gums, esophagus (hoarseness, chronic throat irritation, mouth ulcers, laryngitis, lymph node inflammation and thyroid disorders).

* Tell the truth, listen and be heard.

Food: algae, fruit and blueberries

6th Third-Eye Chakra: brain, nervous system, eyes, ear, nose pineal gland, pituitary gland (brain tumor, effusion, embolism neurological disorders, blindness, deafness, disorders of the entire spine, learning problems and epileptic seizures).

Food: include in your diet tea, chocolate, spices, purple foods, such as red onions, blueberries.

: muscular system, osseous system, skin (depression, chronic exhaustion, extreme sensitivity to light, to sounds and any other environmental factor).

This one doesn't need food to align it as it's nourished by light, air and love, by fasting and detoxification for the elimination of toxins and increase of vital energy.

It's important to mention that emotions play a fundamental role in the health and balance or imbalance of each organ, since negative emotions (sadness, hatred, resentment, and revenge) also acidify our body, lowering its pH level.

Food and good nutrition together with good healthy habits will also help balance these energy points.

To align the Chakras or energy centers we can resort to different tools such as stones, mantras, vibration, meditations and yoga.

All foods have a color, vibration and energy so they also have the ability to harmonize and balance our chakras!

Juice to strengthen lower chakras: root, sacral and solar plexus

Ingredients:

- 1 cup of strawberries
- 1 cup of pineapple
- 1 cup of orange bell peppers
- 1 cup of water

Preparation:

Wash the ingredients, chop the pineapple and peppers, bring everything to the blender along with the water and blend all.

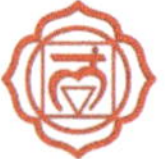  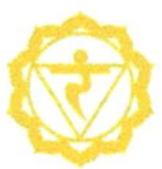

Muladhara   Svadhisthana   Manipura

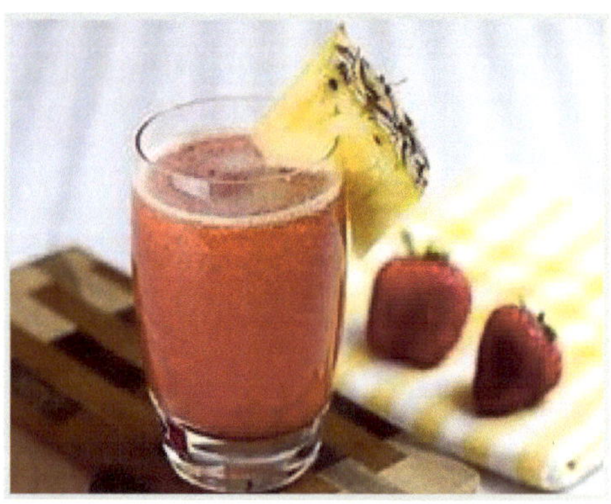

Juice to balance the heart chakra

Ingredients:

- 1 kiwi
- 1 apple
- 1 handful of spinach
- 1 tbsp. of chlorophyll
- 1 cup of water

Preparation:

Wash the ingredients, peel the kiwi, cut the apple into pieces, bring to the blender and add the water and chlorophyll. Blend for a few seconds.

* Take it in the morning or mid afternoon

Anahata

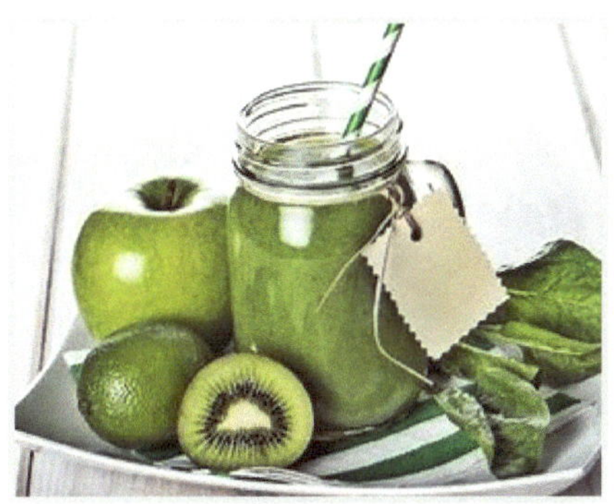

Juice to Balance Upper Chakras: Throat and 3rd Eye

Ingredients:

- 1 cup of blueberries
- 1 cup of black grapes
- 1 plums (seedless)
- 1 small piece of ginger
- 1 cup of water

Preparation:

Wash everything beforehand, peel the ginger, put everything in the blender, add the water and that's it!

*Take it on an empty stomach or mid-afternoon.

 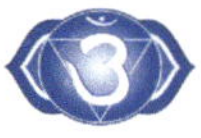

Vishuddha   Ajna

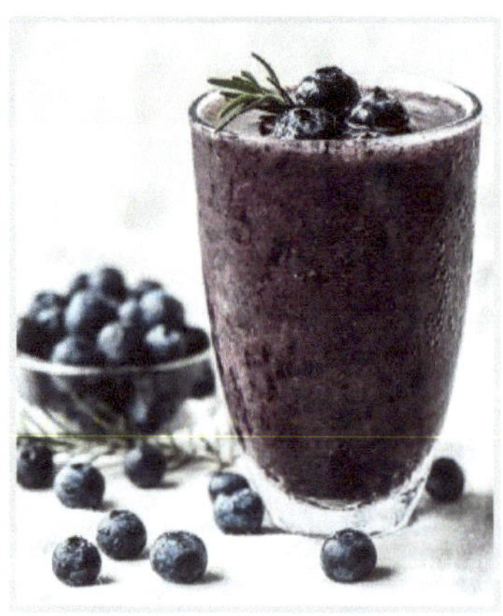

Thank you for coming this far!

I'm very proud of you!

My purpose is to accompany you on this path of learning to choose the best for you and your family, but above all to accompany and inspire you by sharing tools and experiences so that you can improve your health, maintaining healthy habits with a conscious diet full of natural and nutritious foods.

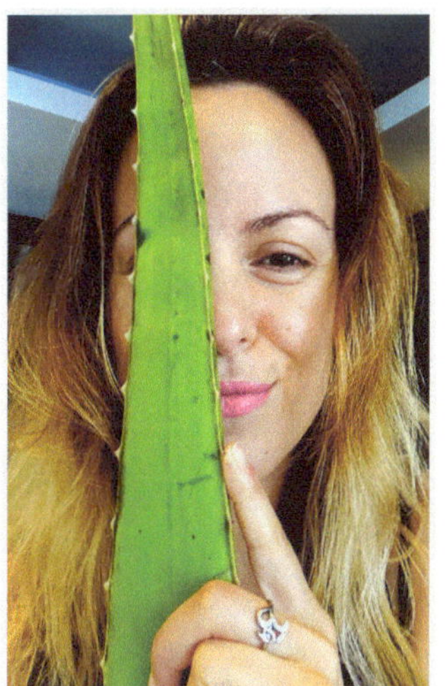

Don't hesitate to contact me!

Find me on social networks, tell me your story
and you will have an ally to maintain a healthy lifestyle!

Instagram: Harmonyhealingwellness
Facebook: harmony healing & wellness
Email: harmonyhealingwellness@gmail.com
Youtube: Harmony Healing & Wellness

Thanks

My infinite thanks to all the people and friends who supported me from the beginning in this wonderful journey and for trusting me and giving me the opportunity to humbly share my knowledge and experiences with all my love.

I want to thank a great friend and very special being for all her love, support and wisdom, which has been an inspiration to me, giving me strength to reinvent myself, guiding me towards my purpose and above all trusting me, thanks @coach_ana.mederos.

I especially want to thank my work team and my husband, my angel, friend and life partner Adrian Antoine, who has encouraged me to carry out this adventure that I had never imagined being able to do, it is something that wouldn't been possible without all his love and unconditional support, giving me strength to be better every day.

Also to my beautiful and talented daughter Jennifer for guiding me with all her love, her patience, her wisdom and photography.

To my father for all the support he gives me day by day, for his teachings, sacrifices and values, thank you dady!

To you, my mom, who accompanies me from heaven, thank you for giving me life and loving me in your own way. God has given us the opportunity to show us that love that we owed ourselves and we needed so much, I love you very much!

And finally, thanks God, to the Universe, to that source of infinite love that shows us the way, as long as we are willing to trust.

www.ingramcontent.com/pod-product-compliance
Lightning Source LLC
Chambersburg PA
CBHW040926110726
48006CB00001B/78